I0053708

THE BOOK OF PROGNOSTICS

Hippocrates of Kos

Translated by: *Francis Adams*
Edited by: *D.P. Curtin*

Dalcassian
Publishing
Company
PHILADELPHIA, PA

The Book of Prognostics

All rights reserved. No part of the material protected by this copyright may be reproduced or utilized in any form, electronic or mechanical, including photocopying, recording or by any information storage and retrieval system, without written permission from the copyright owner.

Library of Congress Cataloging-in-Publication Data

Copyright © 2023 Dalcassian Publishing Co.
All rights reserved.

The Book of Prognostics

Part I

It appears to me a most excellent thing for the physician to cultivate Prognosis; for by foreseeing and foretelling, in the presence of the sick, the present, the past, and the future, and explaining the omissions which patients have been guilty of, he will be the more readily believed to be acquainted with the circumstances of the sick; so that men will have confidence to intrust themselves to such a physician. And he will manage the cure best who has foreseen what is to happen from the present state of matters. For it is impossible to make all the sick well; this, indeed, would have been better than to be able to foretell what is going to happen; but since men die, some even before calling the physician, from the violence of the disease, and some die immediately after calling him, having lived, perhaps, only one day or a little longer, and before the physician could bring his art to counteract the disease; it therefore becomes necessary to know the nature of such affections, how far they are above the powers of the constitution; and, moreover, if there be anything divine in the diseases, and to learn a foreknowledge of this also. Thus a man will be the more esteemed to be a good physician, for he will be the better able to treat those aright who can be saved, having long anticipated everything; and by seeing and announcing beforehand those who will live and those who will die, he will thus escape censure.

Part II

He should observe thus in acute diseases: first, the countenance of the patient, if it be like those of persons in health, and more so, if like itself, for this is the best of all; whereas the most opposite to it is the worst, such as the following; a sharp nose, hollow eyes, collapsed temples; the ears cold, contracted, and their lobes turned out: the skin about the forehead being rough, distended, and parched; the color of the whole face being green, black, livid, or lead-colored. If the countenance be such at the commencement of the disease, and if this cannot be accounted for from the other symptoms, inquiry must be made whether the patient has long wanted sleep; whether his bowels have been very loose; and whether he has suffered from want of food; and if any of these causes be confessed to, the danger is to be reckoned so far less; and it becomes obvious, in the course of a day and a night, whether or not the appearance of the countenance proceeded from these causes. But if none of these be said to exist, if the symptoms do not subside in the aforesaid time, it is to be known for certain that death is at hand. And, also, if the disease be in a more advanced stage either on the third or fourth day, and the countenance be such, the same inquiries as formerly directed are to be made, and the other symptoms are to be noted, those in the whole countenance, those on the body, and those in the eyes; for if they shun the light, or weep involuntarily, or squint, or if the one be less than the other, or if the white of them be red, livid, or has black veins in it; if there be a gum upon the eyes, if they are restless, protruding, or are become very hollow; and if the countenance be squalid and dark, or the color of the whole face be changed-all these are to be reckoned bad and fatal symptoms. The physician should also observe the appearance of the eyes from below the eyelids in sleep; for when a portion of the white appears, owing to the eyelids not being closed together, and when this is not connected with diarrhea or purgation from medicine, or when the patient does not sleep thus from habit, it is to be reckoned an unfavorable and very deadly symptom; but if the eyelid be contracted, livid, or pale, or also the lip, or nose, along with some of the other symptoms, one may know for certain that death is close at hand. It is a mortal symptom, also, when the lips are relaxed, pendent, cold, and blanched.

Part III

It is well when the patient is found by his physician reclining upon either his right or his left side, having his hands, neck, and legs slightly bent, and the whole body lying in a relaxed state, for thus the most of persons in health recline, and these are the best of postures which most resemble those of healthy persons. But to lie upon one's back, with the hands, neck, and the legs extended, is far less favorable. And if the patient incline forward, and sink down to the foot of the bed, it is a still more dangerous symptom; but if he be found with his feet naked and not sufficiently warm, and the hands, neck, and legs tossed about in a disorderly manner and naked, it is bad, for it indicates aberration of intellect. It is a deadly symptom, also, when the patient sleeps constantly with his mouth open, having his legs strongly bent and plaited together, while he lies upon his back; and to lie upon one's belly, when not habitual to the patient to sleep thus while in good health, indicates delirium, or pain in the abdominal regions. And for the patient to wish to sit erect at the acme of a disease is a bad symptom in all acute diseases, but particularly so in pneumonia. To grind the teeth in fevers, when such has not been the custom of the patient from childhood, indicates madness and death, both which dangers are to be announced beforehand as likely to happen; and if a person in delirium do this it is a very deadly symptom. And if the patient had an ulcer previously, or if one has occurred in the course of the disease, it is to be observed; for if the man be about to die the sore will become livid and dry, or yellow and dry before death.

Part IV

Respecting the movement of the hands I have these observations to make: When in acute fevers, pneumonia, phrenitis, or headache, the hands are waved before the face, hunting through empty space, as if gathering bits of straw, picking the nap from the coverlet, or tearing chaff from the wall- all such symptoms are bad and deadly.

Part V

Respiration, when frequent, indicates pain or inflanunation in the parts above the diaphragm: a large respiration performed at a great interval announces delirium; but a cold respiration at nose or mouth is a very fatal symptom. Free respiration is to be looked upon as contributing much to the safety of the patient in all acute diseases, such as fevers, and those complaints which come to a crisis in forty days.

Part VI

Those sweats are the best in all acute diseases which occur on the critical days, and completely carry off the fever. Those are favorable, too, which taking place over the whole body, show that the man is bearing the disease better. But those that do not produce this effect are not beneficial. The worst are cold sweats, confined to the head, face, and neck; these in an acute fever prognosticate death, or in a milder one, a prolongation of the disease; and sweats which occur over the whole body, with the characters of those confined to the neck, are in like manner bad. Sweats attended with a miliary eruption, and taking place about the neck, are bad; sweats in the form of drops and of vapour are good. One ought to know the entire character of sweats, for some are connected with prostration of strength in the body, and some with intensity of the inflammation.

Part VII

That state of the hypochondrium is best when it is free from pain, soft, and of equal size on the right side and the left. But if inflamed, or painful, or distended; or when the right and left sides are of disproportionate sizes;- all these appearances are to be dreaded. And if there be also pulsation in the hypochondrium, it indicates perturbation or delirium; and the physician should examine the eyes of such persons; for if their pupils be in rapid motion, such persons may be expected to go mad. A swelling in the hypochondrium, that is hard and painful, is very bad, provided it occupy the whole hypochondrium; but if it be on either side, it is less dangerous when on the left. Such swellings at the commencement of the disease prognosticate speedy death; but if the fever has passed twenty days, and the swelling has not subsided, it turns to a suppuration. A discharge of blood from the nose occurs to such in the first period, and proves very useful; but inquiry should be made if they have headache or indistinct vision; for if there be such, the disease will be determined thither. The discharge of blood is rather to be expected in those who are younger than thirty-five years. Such swellings as are soft, free from pain, and yield to the finger, occasion more protracted crises, and are less dangerous than the others. But if the fever continue beyond sixty days, without any subsidence of the swelling, it indicates that empyema is about to take place; and a swelling in any other part of the cavity will terminate in like manner. Such, then, as are painful, hard, and large, indicate danger of speedy death; but such as are soft, free of pain, and yield when pressed with the finger, are more chronic than these. Swellings in the belly less frequently form abscesses than those in the hypochondrium; and seldomest of all, those below the navel are converted into suppuration; but you may rather expect a hemorrhage from the upper parts. But the suppuration of all protracted swellings about these parts is to be anticipated. The collections of matter there are to be thus judged of: such as are determined outwards are the best when they are small, when they protrude very much, and swell to a point; such as are large and broad, and which do not swell out to a sharp point, are the worst. Of such as break internally, the best are those which have no external communication, but are covered and indolent; and when the whole place is free from discoloration. That pus is best which is white, homogeneous, smooth, and not at all fetid; the contrary to this is the worst.

Part VIII

All dropsies arising from acute diseases are bad; for they do not remove the fever, and are very painful and fatal. The most of them commence from the flanks and loins, but some from the liver; in those which derive their origin from the flanks and loins the feet swell, protracted diarrhoeas supervene, which neither remove the pains in the flanks and loins, nor soften the belly, but in dropsies which are connected with the liver there is a tickling cough, with scarcely any perceptible expectoration, and the feet swell; there are no evacuations from the bowels, unless such as are hard and forced; and there are swellings about the belly, sometimes on the one side and sometimes on the other, and these increase and diminish by turns.

Part IX

It is a bad symptom when the head, hands, and feet are cold, while the belly and sides are hot; but it is a very good symptom when the whole body is equally hot. The patient ought to be able to turn round easily, and to be agile when raised up; but if he appear heavy in the rest of his body as well as in his hands and feet, it is more dangerous; and if, in addition to the weight, his nails and fingers become livid, immediate death may be anticipated; and if the hands and feet be black it is less dangerous than if they be livid, but the other symptoms must be attended, to; for if he appear to bear the illness well, and if certain of the salutary symptoms appear along with these there may be hope that the disease will turn to a deposition, so that the man may recover; but the blackened parts of the body will drop off. When the testicles and members are retracted upwards, they indicate strong pains and danger of death.

Part X

With regard to sleep- as is usual with us in health, the patient should wake during the day and sleep during the night. If this rule be anywise altered it is so far worse: but there will be little harm provided he sleep in the morning for the third part of the day; such sleep as takes place after this time is more unfavorable; but the worst of all is to get no sleep either night or day; for it follows from this symptom that the insomnolency is connected with sorrow and pains, or that he is about to become delirious.

Part XI

The excrement is best which is soft and consistent, is passed at the hour which was customary to the patient when in health, in quantity proportionate to the ingests; for when the passages are such, the lower belly is in a healthy state. But if the discharges be fluid, it is favorable that they are not accompanied with a noise, nor are frequent, nor in great quantity; for the man being oppressed by frequently getting up, must be deprived of sleep; and if the evacuations be both frequent and large, there is danger of his falling into deliquium animi. But in proportion to the ingesta he should have evacuations twice or thrice in the day, once at night and more copiously in the morning, as is customary with a person in health. The faeces should become thicker when the disease is tending to a crisis; they ought to be yellowish and not very fetid. It is favorable that round worms be passed with the discharges when the disease is tending to a crisis. The belly, too, through the whole disease, should be soft and moderately distended; but excrements that are very watery, or white, or green, or very red, or frothy, are all bad. It is also bad when the discharge is small, and viscid, and white, and greenish, and smooth; but still more deadly appearances are the black, or fatty, or livid, or verdigris-green, or fetid. Such as are of varied characters indicate greater duration of the complaint, but are no less dangerous; such as those which resemble scrapings, those which are bilious, those resembling leeks, and the black; these being sometimes passed together, and sometimes singly. It is best when wind passes without noise, but it is better that flatulence should pass even thus than that it should be retained; and when it does pass thus, it indicates either that the man is in pain or in delirium, unless he gives vent to the wind spontaneously. Pains in the hypochondria, and swellings, if recent, and not accompanied with inflammation, are relieved by borborygmi supervening in the hypochondrium, more especially if it pass off with faeces, urine, and wind; but even although not, it will do good by passing along, and it also does good by descending to the lower part of the belly.

Part XII

The urine is best when the sediment is white, smooth, and consistent during the whole time, until the disease come to a crisis, for it indicates freedom from danger, and an illness of short duration; but if deficient, and if it be sometimes passed clear, and sometimes with a white and smooth sediment, the disease will be more protracted, and not so void of danger. But if the urine be reddish, and the sediment consistent and smooth, the affection, in this case, will be more protracted than the former, but still not fatal. But farinaceous sediments in the urine are bad, and still worse are the leafy; the white and thin are very bad, but the furfuraceous are still worse than these. Clouds carried about in the urine are good when white, but bad if black. When the urine is yellow and thin, it indicates that the disease is unconcocted; and if it (the disease) should be protracted, there maybe danger lest the patient should not hold out until the urine be concocted. But the most deadly of all kinds of urine are the fetid, watery, black, and thick; in adult men and women the black is of all kinds of urine the worst, but in children, the watery. In those who pass thin and crude urine for a length of time, if they have otherwise symptoms of convalescence, an abscess may be expected to form in the parts below the diaphragm. And fatty substances floating on the surface are to be dreaded, for they are indications of melting. And one should consider respecting the kinds of urine, which have clouds, whether they tend upwards or downwards, and upwards or downwards, and the colors which they have and such as fall downwards, with the colors as described, are to be reckoned good and commended; but such as are carried upwards, with the colors as described, are to be held as bad, and are to be distrusted. But you must not allow yourself to be deceived if such urine be passed while the bladder is diseased; for then it is a symptom of the state, not of the general system, but of a particular viscus.

Part XIII

That vomiting is of most service which consists of phlegm and bile mixed together, and neither very thick nor in great quantity; but those vomitings which are more unmixed are worse. But if that which is vomited be of the color of leeks or livid, or black, whatever of these colors it be, it is to be reckoned bad; but if the same man vomit all these colors, it is to be reckoned a very fatal symptom. But of all the vomitings, the livid indicates the danger of death, provided it be of a fetid smell. But all the smells which are somewhat putrid and fetid, are bad in all vomitings.

Part XIV

The expectoration in all pains about the lungs and sides, should be quickly and easily brought up, and a certain degree of yellowness should appear strongly mixed up with the sputum. But if brought up long after the commencement of the pain, and of a yellow or ruddy color, or if it occasions much cough, or be not strongly mixed, it is worse; for that which is intensely yellow is dangerous, but the white, and viscid, and round, do no good. But that which is very green and frothy is bad; but if so intense as to appear black, it is still more dangerous than these; it is dangerous than these; it is bad, if nothing is expectorated, and the lungs discharge nothing, but are gorged with matters which boil (as it were) in the air-passages. It is bad when coryza and sneezing either precede or follow affections of the lungs, but in all other affections, even the most deadly, sneezing is a salutary symptom. A yellow spittle mixed up with not much blood in cases of pneumonia, is salutary and very beneficial if spit up at the commencement of the disease, but if on the seventh day, or still later, it is less favorable. And all sputa are bad which do not remove the pain. But the worst is the black, as has been described. Of all others the sputa which remove the pain are the best.

Part XV

When the pains in these regions do not cease, either with the discharge of the sputa, nor with alvine evacuations, nor from venesection, purging with medicine, nor a suitable regimen, it is to be held that they will terminate in suppurations. Of empyemata such as are spit up while the sputum is still bilious, are very fatal, whether the bilious portion be expectorated separate, or along with the other; but more especially if the empyema begin to advance after this sputum on the seventh day of the disease. It is to be expected that a person with such an expectoration shall die on the fourteenth day, unless something favorable supervene. The following are favorable symptoms: to support the disease easily, to have free respiration, to be free from pain, to have the sputa readily brought up, the whole body to appear equally warm and soft, to have no thirst, the urine, and faeces, sleep, and sweats to be all favorable, as described before; when all these symptoms concur, the patient certainly will not die; but if some of these be present and some not, he will not survive longer than the fourteenth day. The bad symptoms are the opposite of these, namely, to bear the disease with difficulty, respiration large and dense, the pain not ceasing, the sputum scarcely coughed up, strong thirst, to have the body unequally affected by the febrile heat, the belly and sides intensely hot, the forehead, hands, and feet cold; the urine, and excrements, the sleep, and sweats, all bad, agreeably to the characters described above; if such a combination of symptoms accompany the expectoration, the man will certainly die before the fourteenth day, and either on the ninth or eleventh. Thus then one may conclude regarding this expectoration, that it is very deadly, and that the patient will not survive until the fourteenth day. It is by balancing the concomitant symptoms whether good or bad, that one is to form a prognosis; for thus it will most probably prove to be a true one. Most other suppurations burst, some on the twentieth, some on the thirtieth, some on the fortieth, and some as late as the sixtieth day.

Part XVI

One should estimate when the commencement of the suppuration will take place, by calculating from the day on which the patient was first seized with fever, or if he had a rigor, and if he says, that there is a weight in the place where he had pain formerly, for these symptoms occur in the commencement of suppurations. One then may expect the rupture of the abscesses to take place from these times according to the periods formerly stated. But if the empyema be only on either side, one should turn him and inquire if he has pain on the other side; and if the one side be hotter than the other, and when laid upon the sound side, one should inquire if he has the feeling of a weight hanging from above, for if so, the empyema will be upon the opposite side to that on which the weight was felt.

Part XVII

Empyema may be recognized in all cases by the following symptoms: In the first place, the fever does not go off, but is slight during the day, and increases at night, and copious sweats supervene, there is a desire to cough, and the patients expectorate nothing worth mentioning, the eyes become hollow, the cheeks have red spots on them, the nails of the hands are bent, the fingers are hot especially their extremities, there are swellings in the feet, they have no desire of food, and small blisters (phlyctaenae) occur over the body. These symptoms attend chronic empyemata, and may be much trusted to; and such as are of short standing are indicated by the same, provided they be accompanied by those signs which occur at the commencement, and if at the same time the patient has some difficulty of breathing. Whether they will break earlier or later may be determined by these symptoms; if there be pain at the commencement, and if the dyspnoea, cough, and ptyalism be severe, the rupture may be expected in the course of twenty days or still earlier; but if the pain be more mild, and all the other symptoms in proportion, you may expect from these the rupture to be later; but pain, dyspnoea, and ptyalism, must take place before the rupture of the abscess. Those patients recover most readily whom the fever leaves the same day that the abscess bursts,- when they recover their appetite speedily, and are freed from the thirst,- when the alvine discharges are small and consistent, the matter white, smooth, uniform in color, and free of phlegm, and if brought up without pain or strong coughing. Those die whom the fever does not leave, or when appearing to leave them it returns with an exacerbation; when they have thirst, but no desire of food, and there are watery discharges from the bowels; when the expectoration is green or livid, or pituitous and frothy; if all these occur they die, but if certain of these symptoms supervene, and others not, some patients die and some recover, after a long interval. But from all the symptoms taken together one should form a judgment, and so in all other cases.

Part XVIII

When abscesses form about the ears, after peripneumonic affections, or depositions of matter take place in the inferior extremities and end in fistula, such persons recover. The following observations are to be made upon them: if the fever persist, and the pain do not cease, if the expectoration be not normal, and if the alvine discharges be neither bilious, nor free and unmixed; and if the urine be neither copious nor have its proper sediment, but if, on the other hand, all the other salutary symptoms be present, in such cases abscesses may be expected to take place. They form in the inferior parts when there is a collection of phlegm about the hypochondria; and in the upper when the continue soft and free of pain, and when dyspnoea having been present for a certain time, ceases without any obvious cause. All deposits which take place in the legs after severe and dangerous attacks of pneumonia, are salutary, but the best are those which occur at the time when the sputa undergo a change; for if the swelling and pain take place while the sputa are changing from yellow and becoming of a purulent character, and are expectorated freely, under these circumstances the man will recover most favorably and the abscess becoming free of pain, will soon cease; but if the expectoration is not free, and the urine does not appear to have the proper sediment, there is danger lest the limb should be maimed, or that the case otherwise should give trouble. But if the abscesses disappear and go back, while expectoration does not take place, and fever prevails, it is a bad symptom; for there is danger that the man may get into a state of delirium and die. Of persons having empyema after peripneumonic affections, those that are advanced in life run the greatest risk of dying; but in the other kinds of empyema younger persons rather die. In cases of empyema treated by the cautery or incision, when the matter is pure, white, and not fetid, the patient recovers; but if of a bloody and dirty character, he dies.

Part XIX

Pains accompanied with fever which occur about the loins and lower parts, if they attack the diaphragm, and leave the parts below, are very fatal. Wherefore one ought to pay attention to the other symptoms, since if any unfavorable one supervene, the case is hopeless; but if while the disease is determined to the diaphragm, the other symptoms are not bad, there is great reason to expect that it will end in empyema. When the bladder is hard and painful, it is an extremely bad and mortal symptom, more especially in cases attended with continued fever; for the pains proceeding from the bladder alone are to kill the patient; and at such a time the bowels are not moved, or the discharges are hard and forced. But urine of a purulent character, and having a white and smooth sediment, relieves the patient. But if no amendment takes place in the characters of the urine, nor the bladder become soft, and the fever is of the continual type, it may be expected that the patient will die in the first stages of the complaint. This form attacks children more especially, from their seventh to their fifteenth year.

Part XX

Fevers come to a crisis on the same days as to number on which men recover and die. For the mildest class of fevers, and those originating with the most favorable symptoms, cease on the fourth day or earlier; and the most malignant, and those setting in with the most dangerous symptoms, prove fatal on the fourth day or earlier. The first class of them as to violence ends thus: the second is protracted to the seventh day, the third to the eleventh, the fourth to the fourteenth, the fifth to the seventeenth, and the sixth to the twentieth. Thus these periods from the most acute disease ascend by fours up to twenty. But none of these can be truly calculated by whole days, for neither the year nor the months can be numbered by entire days. After these in the same manner, according to the same progression, the first period is of thirty-four days, the second of forty days, and the third of sixty days. In the commencement of these it is very difficult to determine those which will come to a crisis after a long interval; for these beginnings are very similar, but one should pay attention from the first day, and observe further at every additional tetrad, and then one cannot miss seeing how the disease will terminate. The constitution of quartans is agreeable to the same order. Those which will come to a crisis in the shortest space of time, are the easiest to be judged of; for the differences of them are greatest from the commencement, thus those who are going to recover breathe freely, and do not suffer pain, they sleep during the night, and have the other salutary symptoms, whereas those that are to die have difficult respiration, are delirious, troubled with insomnolency, and have other bad symptoms. Matters being thus, one may conjecture, according to the time, and each additional period of the diseases, as they proceed to a crisis. And in women, after parturition, the crises proceed agreeably to the same ratio.

Part XXI

Strong and continued headaches with fever, if any of the deadly symptoms be joined to them, are very fatal. But if without such symptoms the pain be prolonged beyond twenty days, a discharge of blood from the nose or some abscess in the inferior parts may be anticipated; but while the pain is recent, we may expect in like manner a discharge of blood from the nose, or a suppuration, especially if the pain be seated above the temples and forehead; but the hemorrhage is rather to be looked for in persons younger than thirty years, and the suppuration in more elderly persons.

Part XXII

Acute pain of the ear, with continual and strong fever, is to be dreaded; for there is danger that the man may become delirious and die. Since, then, this is a hazardous spot, one ought to pay particular attention to all these symptoms from the commencement. Younger persons die of this disease on the seventh day, or still earlier, but old persons much later; for the fevers and delirium less frequently supervene upon them, and on that account the ears previously come to a suppuration, but at these periods of life, relapses of the disease coming on generally prove fatal. Younger persons die before the ear suppurates; only if white matter run from the ear, there may be hope that a younger person will recover, provided any other favorable symptom be combined.

Part XXIII

Ulceration of the throat with fever, is a serious affection, and if any other of the symptoms formerly described as being bad, be present, the physician ought to announce that his patient is in danger. Those quinsies are most dangerous, and most quickly prove fatal, which make no appearance in the fauces, nor in the neck, but occasion very great pain and difficulty of breathing; these induce suffocation on the first day, or on the second, the third, or the fourth. Such as, in like manner, are attended with pain, are swelled up, and have redness (erythema) in the throat, are indeed very fatal, but more protracted than the former, provided the redness be great. Those cases in which both the throat and the neck are red, are more protracted, and certain persons recover from them, especially if the neck and breast be affected with erythema, and the erysipelas be not determined inwardly. If neither the erysipelas disappear on the critical day, nor any abscess form outwardly, nor any pus be spit up, and if the patient fancy himself well, and be free from pain, death, or a relapse of the erythema is to be apprehended. It is much less hazardous when the swelling and redness are determined outwardly; but if determined to the lungs, they superinduce delirium, and frequently some of these cases terminate in empyema. It is very dangerous to cut off or scarify enlarged uvulae while they and red and large, for inflammations and hemorrhages supervene; but one should try to reduce such swellings by some other means at this season. When the whole of it is converted into an abscess, which is called Uva, or when the extremity of the variety called Columella is larger and round, but the upper part thinner, at this time it will be safe to operate. But it will be better to open the bowels gently before proceeding to the operation, if time will permit, and the patient be not in danger of being suffocated.

Part XXIV

When the fevers cease without any symptoms of resolution occurring, and not on the critical days, in such cases a relapse may be anticipated. When any of the fevers is protracted, although the man exhibits symptoms of recovery, and there is no longer pain from any inflammation, nor from any other visible cause, in such a case a deposit, with swelling and pain, may be expected in some one of the joints, and not improbably in those below. Such deposits occur more readily and in less time to persons under thirty years of age; and one should immediately suspect the formation of such a deposit, if the fever be protracted beyond twenty days; but to aged persons these less seldom happen, and not until the fever be much longer protracted. Such a deposit may be expected, when the fever is of a continual type, and that it will pass into a quartan, if it become intermittent, and its paroxysms come on in an irregular manner, and if in this form it approach autumn. As deposits form most readily in persons below thirty years of age, so quartans most commonly occur to persons beyond that age. It is proper to know that deposits occur most readily in winter, that then they are most protracted, but are less given to return. Whoever, in a fever that is not of a fatal character, says that he has pain in his head, and that something dark appears to be before his eyes, and that he has pain at the stomach, will be seized with vomiting of bile; but if rigor also attack him, and the inferior parts of the hypochondrium are cold, vomiting is still nearer at hand; and if he eat or drink anything at such a season, it will be quickly vomited. In these cases, when the pain commences on the first day, they are particularly oppressed on the fourth and the fifth; and they are relieved on the seventh, but the greater part of them begin to have pain on the third day, and are most especially tossed on the fifth, but are relieved on the ninth or eleventh; but in those who begin to have pains on the fifth day, and other matters proceed properly with them, the disease comes to a crisis on the fourteenth day. But when in such a fever persons affected with headache, instead of having a dark appearance before their eyes, have dimness of vision, or flashes of light appear before their eyes, and instead of pain at the pit of the stomach, they have in their hypochondrium a fullness stretching either to the right or left side, without either pain or inflammation, a hemorrhage from the nose is to be expected in such a case, rather than a vomiting. But it is in young persons particularly that the hemorrhage is to be expected, for in persons beyond the age of thirty-five, vomiting are rather to be anticipated. Convulsions occur to children if acute fever be present, and the belly be they cannot sleep, are agitated, and moan, and change color, and become green, livid, or ruddy. These complaints occur most readily to children which are very young up to their seventh year; older children and adults are not equally liable to be seized with convulsions in fevers, unless some of the strongest and worst symptoms precede, such as those which occur in frenzy. One must judge of children as of others, which will die and which recover, from the whole of the symptoms, as they have been specially described. These things I say respecting acute diseases, and the affections which spring from them.

Part XXV

He who would correctly beforehand those that will recover, and those that will die, and in what cases the disease will be protracted for many days, and in what cases for a shorter time, must be able to form a judgment from having made himself acquainted with all the symptoms, and estimating their powers in comparison with one another, as has been described, with regard to the others, and the urine and sputa, as when the patient coughs up pus and pus and bile together. One ought also to consider promptly the influx of epidemical diseases and the constitution of the season. One should likewise be well acquainted with the particular signs and the other symptoms, and not be ignorant how that, in every year, and at every season, bad symptoms prognosticate ill, and favorable symptoms good, since the aforesaid symptoms appear to have held true in Libya, in Delos, and in Scythia, from which it may be known that, in the same regions, there is no difficulty in attaining a knowledge of many more things than these; if having learned them, one knows also how to judge and reason correctly of them. But you should not complain because the name of any disease may happen not to be described here, for you may know all such as come to a crisis in the aforementioned times, by the same symptoms.

www.ingramcontent.com/pod-product-compliance
Lightning Source LLC
Chambersburg PA
CBHW071534210326
41597CB00018B/2992